362-3
362.3.081.
42
P

AF746766

Bel
Thi
below.
made be

27. MAR 86
24. MAR 86
19. MAY 86
13. MAY 86
23. 87
27. FEB 87
1987
11 NOV 1987
10 NOV 1987
21 APR 198
10 APR 1989

Learning to care for MENTALLY HANDICAPPED PEOPLE

Val Pounds
RNMS

Manager, Style Acre, Wallingford
formerly Senior Nursing Officer
and Assistant Director of Nursing,
Wayland Hospital, Bradfield

HODDER AND STOUGHTON
LONDON SYDNEY AUCKLAND TORONTO

11 FEB 1986

LEARNING TO CARE SERIES

General Editors

JEAN HEATH, BA, SRN, SCM, CERT ED
English National Board Learning Resources Unit, Sheffield

SUSAN E. NORMAN, SRN, DN CERT, RNT
Senior Tutor, The Nightingale School, West Lambeth Health Authority

---

Titles in this series include:

Learning to Care for Elderly People
L. THOMAS
Learning to Care in the Community
P. TURTON and J. ORR
Learning to Care on the Medical Ward
A. MATTHEWS
Learning to Care on the ENT Ward
D. STOKES
Learning to Care on the Gynaecology Ward
W. SIMONS

British Library Cataloguing in Publication Data

Pounds, Val
Learning to care for mentally handicapped people.—(Learning to care series)
1. Handicapped—Care and treatment
I. Title
362.4 HV1568

ISBN 0 340 38104 3

DUNDEE COLLEGE OF TECHNOLOGY LIBRARY

First published 1985
Copyright © 1985 V. Pounds

All rights reserved. No part of this publication may be reproduced or transmitted in any form or by any means, electronic or mechanical, including photocopy, recording or any information storage or retrieval system, without permission in writing from the publisher, or under licence from the Copyright Licensing Agency Limited. Further details of such licences (for reprographic reproduction) may be obtained from the Copyright Licensing Agency Limited, of 19 Bedford Square, London WC1.

Typeset in 10/11 pt Trump Mediaeval by Rowland Phototypesetting Ltd, Bury St Edmunds, Suffolk

Printed in Great Britain for Hodder and Stoughton Educational, a division of Hodder and Stoughton Ltd, Mill Road, Dunton Green, Sevenoaks, Kent TN13 2YD, by Richard Clay (The Chaucer Press) Ltd, Bungay, Suffolk.

Editors' Foreword

In most professions there is a traditional gulf between theory and its practice, and nursing is no exception. The gulf is perpetuated when theory is taught in a theoretical setting and practice is taught by the practitioner.

This inherent gulf has to be bridged by students of nursing, and publication of this series is an attempt to aid such bridge building.

It aims to help relate theory and practice in a meaningful way whilst underlining the importance of the person being cared for.

It aims to introduce students of nursing to some of the more common problems found in each new area of experience in which they will be asked to work.

It aims to de-mystify some of the technical language they will hear, putting it in context, giving it meaning and enabling understanding.

Preface

Florence Nightingale said of the Student Nurse: 'I do not pretend to teach her – I ask her to teach herself, and for this purpose, I venture to give her some hints.'

Likewise, the information in the following chapters is meant to supply the Student Nurse with some background knowledge and practical examples which will hopefully stimulate self-tuition and formulation of opinion.

CONTENTS

1 Introduction

So you want to be a nurse for mentally handicapped people. First of all the role of a nurse in this field must be clarified, because it is far removed from the traditional image of bedpans, thermometers and operations! It is argued that the title 'nurse' is inappropriate, and it may well be that in time to come, that title will be changed. We tend to do a lot of title changing in mental handicap.

Over the years we have dispensed with words like 'idiot', 'imbecile', 'asylum', 'mental deficiency', 'mental subnormality', and many others, in a perpetual attempt to remove the stigma which inevitably becomes associated with words describing a low intelligence.

There has been, for several years now, a growing move away from the 'nurse' concept in mental handicap. After all, mental handicap is not an 'illness', although one could argue that certain conditions are treatable, i.e. cretinism, phenylketonuria. With these very few exceptions, it is not treatable, clinically, but those with mental handicap *are* 'trainable'. Therefore, those working with them are possibly 'teachers' rather than nurses. There is another school of thought, which advocates the title 'carers' – a rather ambiguous term. Does it mean we 'care about' or 'care for'? If we care *for*, then we are in some respects returning to the traditional nurse role. Perhaps it would be useful to look at mentally handicapped people in very broad, basic terms, to decide exactly what their needs are, before we decide what it is we are required to do for, to, or with them.

Legal definition of mental handicap: Arrested or incomplete development of the mind

Basically, the mentally handicapped are *people* – like everyone else. They have the four basic physical functions as we do:

Breathing
Eating
Excreting
Sleeping

These four component parts of the human being are common to us all, including mentally handicapped people. Any other physical, mental or spiritual facets to our make-up are arbitrary. The incidence of mental handicap is one in a thousand of the population in Britain, probably as many as in any other range of intelligence if broken down into grades.

My colleagues talk a lot about 'normalisation' for the mentally handicapped. I suggest that mentally handicapped people *are* normal in principle.

They may lack a degree of initiative and intuition – the essential elements of most of our characters, which motivate us to organise our lives. Maybe it is 'prompting' that they need from us most.

Think about your own life style for a moment. Below there is a list of key words which it is useful to think about, in relation to your own life style, and that of the mentally handicapped person. There may be a vast difference in some areas. What you need to think about is, 'Is the difference necessary?' Do they make the same decisions, choices and preferences? If not, why not? These are questions you will repeatedly ask yourself throughout your training.

Hopefully, you will have escaped the institutions which functioned like factories, giving little opportunity for anyone to make a choice about anything. I once heard someone describing his first and only visit to one of these institutions, where he found the habits

KEY WORDS:

Think about each word/topic and rate the difference it means in your own life style and that of a mentally handicapped person. Then consider why.

Clothes	Choice; Colour; Style; Where bought
Food	Likes/Dislikes; Meal times; Menu; Snacks
Privacy	Own bedroom; Bathroom; Toilet
Money	How much; Who holds; Spent on
Holidays	Where to go; Who to go with
Hobbies	Gardening; Knitting; Tennis; Disco; Bingo
Work	Job availability; Training; Hours of work; Wages
Bed	Bedtime; Tea in bed; Get up time
Television	Choice of station and programme; Switch-off time
Leisure time	How spent; Proportion of time
Books	What type
Conversation	About what; Who with; When
Eating out	Where; Who with; When; What food

of the inmates quite intriguing. Among his observations about the mentally handicapped was the outrageous assumption – 'and they all take sugar'. So would we, if all our lives sugar had been added to the family teapot!

Definition of mental impairment: In addition to incomplete or arrested development, there is significant impairment of intelligence and social functioning with abnormally aggressive or irresponsible conduct

I suggest that we, the carers, teachers, nurses – whatever – actually manufacture abnormal characteristics in the mentally handicapped by the way we organise their lives. These abnormal characteristics are then very often considered symptoms of their condition. Characteristics such as 'all taking sugar' are perhaps not so very important, but other social behaviours which are manufactured *are*. Many mentally handicapped people may be labelled 'aggressive', 'disruptive', 'destructive', etc., because of the circumstances imposed upon them – we do them a great injustice.

I hope that you, as a newcomer, will think very carefully about this, and not allow yourself to be drawn along with the crowd, taking for granted every fact that presents itself. There are seldom enough staff in hospitals, and the environment is often not wholly conducive to caring for the mentally handicapped person. What you must resolve to do is to make sure that the very best is being done with the resources available. Do not fall into the trap of using less than ideal facilities and circumstances as an excuse for not delivering the best possible service, given the constraints. Apathy becomes a habit all too easily.

As in most professions, mental handicap nursing is not without its technical jargon. You will hear many phrases such as 'crisis intervention', 'goal planning', etc. They may sound very intriguing, but there is nothing mystical about them. Most are simple skills we use in everyday life, usually subconsciously. In caring for mentally handicapped people, we need to consciously develop these skills. For example, we all 'deal' with minor aggression and anti-social behaviour in 'normal' people – often without realising it. Aggression or anti-social behaviour may be more pronounced in the mentally handicapped person, and therefore we have to consciously learn and plan our responses. A successful nurse in mental handicap is one who has a stable, tolerant personality, lots of good common sense, and a continuing commitment to develop her skills.

The modern day philosophy of care advocates that all mentally handicapped people are entitled to the same rights as normal people. That includes the right to work, vote, live like others in the community, marry, procreate, and receive benefits and services which are available to other people. However, 'other people' have responsibilities as well as rights, and as far as possible the mentally handicapped person should have responsibilities too.

This is a whole new concept, far removed from the custodial and protective philosophies of the past which, whilst possibly safer and more comfortable, caused the mentally handicapped person to be devalued as a human being in society. To achieve the rightful esteem of these under-endowed people, the nurse must act as advocate, and prompt and assist the handicapped person to develop their individual personality and to assert themselves in the way that other people do.

In the chapters which follow, we will be paying attention also to the families of the mentally handicapped person. It is often the case that other members of the family, or the family as a whole, require support and assistance to come to terms and adjust to what they see as shameful, degrading or intolerable circumstances. 'Why did *we* have to have a less than perfect child?', 'Whose fault is it?', 'We must be abnormal to produce such a child'. These are all questions which you will hear many parents exclaim. You will witness siblings displaying reactionary behaviour, and leaving home early out of embarrassment or disgust. You will meet many strained or broken marriages brought about by the existence of a mentally handicapped child. You will also be aware of a few families who are brought closer together because of the dependent mentally handicapped child. You will certainly have to learn to deal with distress, tragedy, and grief. The families of the mentally handicapped are often far more vulnerable than the handicapped member. Parents are usually comforted to know that there is a name for, and a reason why, their offspring is not as other children.

There are a number of known causes of mental handicap, and still a few obscure incidences. I do not propose to give a text book summary of the causes and syndromes known, as there are already many useful books in which this detailed information can be found, but a very condensed chart of common causes is given at the end of this chapter.

The majority of mentally handicapped people come into the 'unknown origin' category. Knowing the cause and etiology does not necessarily help the nurse to care for her patient, but studies over the years have, of course, brought about a few 'treatments' and considerable prevention of mental handicap by way of genetic counselling.

Epilepsy is often associated with mental handicap, although it is frequently present in people of normal intelligence. There have been numerous beliefs over the years about the personality and behaviour of epileptics. Whilst there is some justification for acknowledging that some epileptics display unstable temperament, moodiness, aggressiveness, and untruthfulness, it is unfair and unwise to suppose that these characteristics are necessarily present in all people with epilepsy. As with mental handicap generally, philosophies about the lifestyle of the epileptic have changed dramatically.

It used to be customary to protect the epileptic person from virtually all the elements of life. They were not allowed to sleep in a normal height bed, in case they fell out in a fit, handle any electrical appliance, climb steps or stairs, or bathe unsupervised. Food was minced in case they had a fit and choked on solid food, and 'black jack' was handed out every Friday night to ensure regular bowel evacuation. All sharp instruments were forbidden, and even the most capable epileptic in a subnormality hospital was subjected to using a spoon to eat, as knives and forks were thought to be a risk.

Today, people with epilepsy, be they mentally handicapped or not, are encouraged to live as normally as possible. Avoidance of activities involving risk sometimes induces the kind of anti-social behaviour previously attributed to them. Modern drug therapy has reduced the incidence of epileptic fits for most people, but the nurse should be especially vigilant to the side effects of long-term administration. In some cases, the side effects can be as unpleasant as the seizures.

Common side effects:
Drowsiness
Gum atrophy
Dry mouth
Tremor
Skin irritation

Modern philosophy suggests that a variety of services and facilities should be available to provide a comprehensive pattern of care for the mentally handicapped – hospital being the least desirable environment on a long-term basis. Therefore, it is more appropriate to illustrate case studies from different models of care, rather than confine the following chapters to the various types of hospital wards only.

Mental handicap nursing is rapidly becoming a 'mobile service'. Traditionally, the patient came to the nurse or hospital. Today, the nurse (and all support services) go to the patient wherever possible. Very often the problem is in the home, and taking the handicapped person into hospital will achieve little. The nurse has to assess the problem in the handicapped person's usual environment and,

Refer to: *Care in the Community*. DHSS HC (81) 9.

with the involvement of other professionals if appropriate, will devise a programme or plan to alleviate or lessen the problem. This is achieved with the total involvement of the family, who should understand the explanation and learn to respond appropriately when the care plan is implemented and demonstrated in the home where the family lives.

However, whilst the emphasis is on alternative forms of care, we should not underestimate the role that the traditional hospital plays. It is unfortunate that hospitals are often thought of as the 'last resort' or 'the dumping ground' for those seemingly hopeless cases who do not respond to other forms of care, or who prove too disruptive to manage in integrated environments.

Other agencies:
Social services
Voluntary sector
Private sector

Other disciplines:
Psychiatrist
Psychologist
Physiotherapist
Occupational therapist
Social worker
Speech therapist

You will learn that mental handicap care is very much a team effort. There are many people and agencies involved, and they all have a part to play. Although nurses are the majority group, the role of the nurse is perhaps less well defined than other professionals. It is a mistake for nurses to see themselves as the assistants to the other disciplines involved. It is suggested that this only happens when the nurse has no positive contribution to make, no innovative ideas of her own, and does not recognise her own professional expertise. Make sure that you subject yourself to self-analysis frequently. Review the way you handle problems – with colleagues as well as patients – to ensure that you make a positive and therapeutic contribution.

During your training, you will be working alongside school teachers, social workers, psychologists, psychiatrists, and many other people involved with mental handicap and you will be allocated to a variety of departments and establishments other than hospital wards. You will observe different attitudes of staff, and learn to form your own opinions with experience about what constitutes the 'right attitude'.

Care has been taken in selecting the case studies which follow not to create an over-pessimistic or optimistic view. Not all cases are success stories, or likewise, failure stories. The nurse will be exposed to both, but no cause is ever completely lost, and she must be resilient and resourceful in the face of seemingly impossible problems. There is great reward and satisfaction in seeing development and achievement in the majority of people she will care for.

The nurse must be firmly committed to improving the quality of life and the individual self-help skills of mentally handicapped people, and assisting them to live an ordinary life.

The characters and details in the following case studies have been deliberately altered to avoid easy identification, and in some instances, features which are normally present in a particular condition have been included to give a more typical clinical example.

Normalisation philosophy

It is recognised that mentally handicapped people have the same human value as other people in society. They have the same rights, and as far as possible, the same responsibilities as other people. In addition, they have a right to receive the attention and assistance of all professional services, to enable them to achieve as normal a life as possible.

The nurse's role in the field of mental handicap is to skilfully facilitate all the assistance the mentally handicapped person and their family require, and to extend to the full potential each person's individual 'living' skills. The nurse should show respect for the individual personalities and characteristics of people with mental handicap, and set an example of acceptance.

SOME CAUSES OF MENTAL HANDICAP:
Primary/genetic causes

Condition	*Possible cause*	*Common symptoms*
Down's syndrome	Extra chromosome in pair 21	Short stature; well spaced slanting eyes; epicanthic fold; large roughened tongue; palmar crease; congenital heart abnormalities; circulatory disturbances; chest infections
Sturge–Weber syndrome	May be associated with trisomy 22	Half face, neck and upper chest are 'port-wine stained' with a naevus; hemiparesis on opposite side of body; epilepsy
Tuberous sclerosis	Single dominant gene of poor penetrance	1 Mental handicap 2 Epilepsy 3 Adenoma sebaceum (butterfly facial rash)
Phenylketonuria	Metabolic disorder; single recessive gene	If not arrested – epilepsy; mental handicap; fair hair and complexion; blue eyes (lack of pigmentation). Treatable with phenylalanine-free diet – early detection is essential
Gargoylism	Single recessive or sex-linked gene	Characteristic facial appearance resembling a gargoyle; large head; frontal bossing; prominent supraorbital ridges; depressed bridge of nose; coarse bushy eyebrows; large fissured tongue; short in stature and limbs; enlarged liver and spleen
Cretinism	Genetic deficiency of thyroid gland	Stunted growth; apathy; enlarged protruding tongue; yellowish wrinkled skin; extended abdomen – umbilical hernia; scanty hair; subnormal body temperature; treatable with extract of thyroid. Early detection essential

Secondary causes

Condition	*Possible cause*	*Common symptoms*
Rubella syndrome	Maternal rubella in first three months of pregnancy	Microcephaly; blindness; deafness; severe mental handicap
Toxoplasmosis	Maternal protozoal infection contracted from domestic pets and farm animals	Micro- or hydrocephaly; spastic deformities; epilepsy; enlargement of liver and spleen
Encephalitis	Virus	Hemiplegia; athetoid movements; epilepsy; aphasia; ataxia; personality disorders
Anoxic amentia	Deprivation of oxygen at birth; infantile gastroenteritis	Hemiparesis; epilepsy; varying degree of mental handicap
Traumatic amentia	Severe trauma during pregnancy or birth; excessive radiation during pregnancy; Rhesus incompatibility	Microcephaly; plegia; epilepsy; severe mental handicap
Deprivation amentia	1 Nutritional deficiencies 2 Sensory isolation (deafness/ blindness) 3 Environmental	Varied symptoms

2 Life begins at 70

HISTORY

Edna Briggs was born illegitimately in 1910 to a young girl of simple intelligence who was 'in-service' to a very respected family in Bristol. Her mother was immediately dismissed from her position, and the next few years of Edna's life are somewhat obscure, but at the age of six years, she was committed, with her mother, to the workhouse for stealing food. Edna spent the next 60 years of her life in institutions of one sort or another. There was no good reason for this. She just had nowhere to go, and her mother, who was her only known family, died whilst they were still in the workhouse.

In 1964 Edna was 'privileged' to be allowed to enter private employment, working out from the hospital for a local lady as a housemaid, for which she received five shillings a week. Her employer was very good to Edna, and lavished presents on her at Christmas and holiday times, but did not accept that Edna could have any real need or understanding of regular remuneration for her duties. Edna did not mind this exploitation, and looked upon her employer as the only 'family' she had. One can imagine her distress when the lady of the house moved away, and Edna's employment and attachment came to an end.

At this time Edna was living on a hospital ward with nine other elderly ladies with mild mental handicap. This was a four-star environment compared with the institutional conditions she had endured over the years, but Edna often talked about 'going outside' to live. The staff on the ward felt that Edna's life-experiences could not possibly have equipped her to make such a decision, or understand what 'life outside' was all about.

However, in 1981, when a place became available in the Core and Cluster model serving her hospital, she expressed a desire to leave. A full assessment was made of her self-help and social skills, which were, surprisingly, quite high. Edna had been attending the Training Department, where she had very quickly and easily learned the art of simple cooking, shopping, laundering, etc.

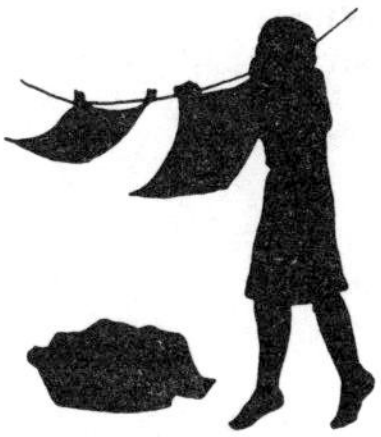

At the age of 70, her potential for development was not thought very encouraging, but it was finally decided that Edna should be given a month's trial in the Core House.

The Core and Cluster model of care

There are several varieties of the Core and Cluster theme, all originating from the Encor Model in Nebraska. It consists of a 'Core House' which is a large staffed house, where clients are admitted, assessed, and given appropriate training in independence skills. This house, although serving as the management/administrative base for the cluster houses, must essentially be as homely as possible. This is where institutional habits will be replaced by more acceptable and individual characteristics. This is not always easy to achieve, and very careful assessment, planning and evaluation (which together form the nursing process) are essential.

The staff are a closely-knit team, doing a highly skilled job – teaching and helping people to live normally. Careful development programmes are devised for each individual client. Seemingly outrageous practices, compared with hospital regimes, go on – clients are taught to hold and administer their own drugs, hold their own bank books, launder their own clothes, etc. These are all very important preparations for moving on to one of the Cluster Houses.

Core and Cluster model showing the variety of living facilities and services which clients are made aware of and encouraged to use appropriately

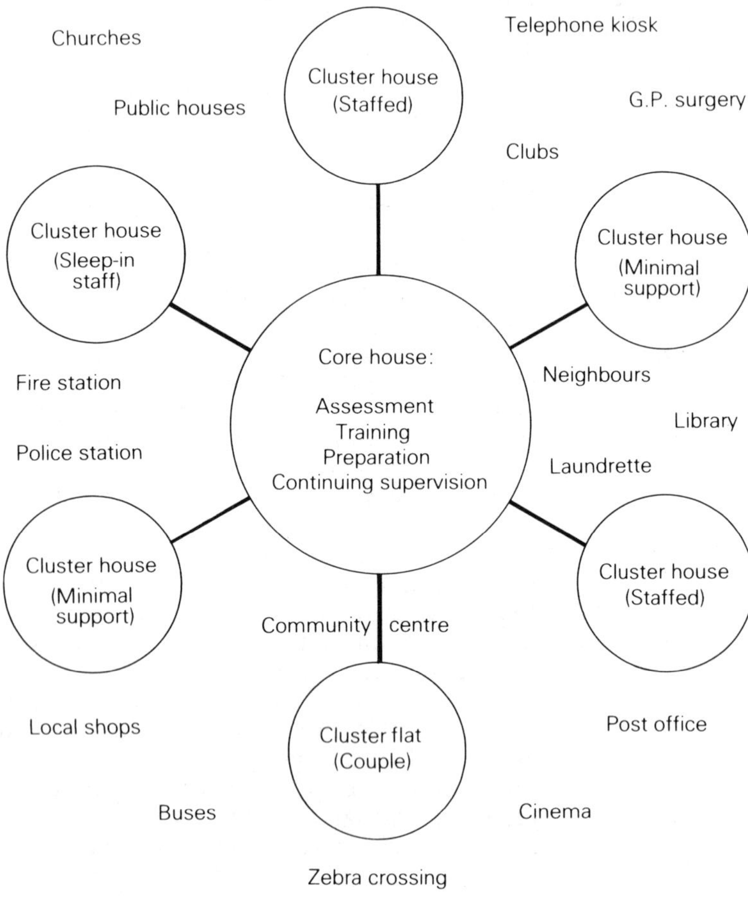

The 'Cluster' is a number of ordinary, domestic-type houses within a ⅔ mile radius of the core. Groups of three or four mentally handicapped people live in each house, as independently as possible, but with whatever level of support is required from the staff of the core.

At this stage, they are able to draw DHSS benefits, and contribute equally to the rent, telephone bill, food, etc. They will be encouraged and assisted to seek open employment, or daytime activity suitable to their age, abilities, and needs.

It is likely that the level of support required will be different in each house. Some cluster houses will require full-time staff in-put.

All services which are available to ordinary people should be available to the cluster residents, and they will be registered with a local G.P., draw their benefits from the local Post Office, use the local laundrette, shops, cafes, pubs, churches and social centres. If operated successfully, the cluster houses, and residents, will blend in with the local community without appearing conspicuous in any way. It is important that the cluster houses are not next door to each other to avoid saturation of a locality with people who quickly become obvious in large numbers as 'different'.

EDNA'S TRIAL MONTH

Edna soon settled down in the core house, and adjusted to her new-found freedom with surprising confidence. It soon became obvious that there was little the staff could teach her in the way of living skills. All she required was the opportunity to practise them. At 70 years of age, she relished the walk to the town to shop or have tea in the corner cafe. She made new acquaintances, budgeted her money extremely well, and wrote long sensible accounts of her new lifestyle to all her friends back at the hospital.

Edna and three other clients were selected to move into a cluster house together. It was the first occupation of this particular house, which was detached, on a private housing estate, and had been standing empty for some time. The introduction of the group on to this estate was very carefully planned. It was recognised that the neighbours were not impressed with the neglected appearance of the house, which had grass and weeds growing up over the windows and covering the paths. It was therefore assumed that they would be pleased to find the house being put into order before occupation. The staff took two of the four prospective residents to the house each day, and they set about clearing the garden, cleaning the windows, and generally tidying up. It was not long before the neighbours were handing cups of tea over the fence to this hard-working group, without realising that two of them would be their new neighbours. And so it was that the group was gradually introduced, and by the time the house was fit for occupation, the neighbours were quite confident that the group was very capable of being 'good neighbours'.

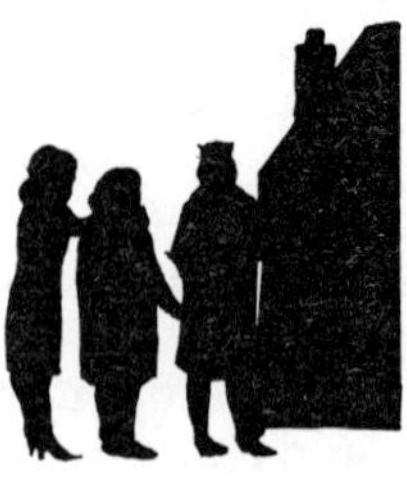

In August, they moved in. They had chosen their own bedroom furniture and colour schemes, and the house was by then decorated throughout and the garden immaculate. The two men in the group made themselves responsible for the garden and the shopping, and kept their own bedrooms clean. Edna and the other lady did most of the cooking and general housework. Before long, they had acquired a cat, a budgerigar, and two goldfish which they cherished with tender loving care.

Edna's basic assessment

	Unaided	*Aided*	*Action/remarks*
Daily living skills			
Washes	√		
Dresses	√		
Makes bed	√		
Clothes care		√	Practice with washing machine and iron
Hair care	√		Goes to hairdresser
Nail care		√	Practice with nail clippers on toes
Travels alone		√	Familiarisation with bus stops
Shops	√		
Uses telephone		√	Hearing impairment – amplifier
Simple cooking	√		
Social skills			
Makes friends	√		
Makes conversation	√		
Acceptable behaviour	√		
Intellectual skills			
Reads	√		Eyes re-tested
Writes	√		
Money values	√		Instruction on use of Post Office Savings Book

CARE PLAN

for Edna

Problem and aim: She is disorientated in town and needs to be familiarised with local shops, direction, etc.
Nursing care: Escort her into town, encouraging her to lead the way. Practise touring the shops and finding the Post Office, bus stops, etc. Arrange to meet her at a familiar shop entrance and ask her to direct you to various places.

Problem and aim: She cannot operate a coin laundrette and needs to be shown how.
Nursing care: Go with her to the local laundrette and prompt her through the procedure step by step. This may have to be repeated on many occasions. Reduce prompting as she becomes more confident and proficient.

Problem and aim: She cannot hear a doorbell or telephone and needs her hearing supplemented.
Nursing care: Arrange a hearing assessment and follow-up applications for aids, e.g. amplifier on telephone, re-actor lights on doorbell and telephone. Encourage other members of the group to recognise her hearing difficulty and make sure that she is not left out of conversations.

All went well, and Edna's group was a credit to the staff who had prepared and supported them. But at 70, how long could it last? Edna became noticeably deaf, and could not hear the telephone or the doorbell. She also began to be isolated from the group, spending a lot of time walking in town on her own, or in her bedroom because she could not hear and join in the conversation. She compensated by writing long daily letters to all her former friends at the hospital, with whom she never lost contact. The staff began to feel that perhaps Edna had been too old after all, and that it was only a matter of time before she would have to be re-admitted. Fortunately, after long discussions and debate, it was decided that Edna's hearing impairment made her no different from ordinary deaf people, and she was taken to the audio clinic. After a complete hearing assessment and home visit, Edna was fitted with a hearing aid, and household gadgets were supplied by the Hearing Centre which included flashing lights attached to the doorbell and telephone, and an individual amplifier fitted to the television, to allow the other members of the household to enjoy normal volume.

Edna's temporary isolation was not instantly overcome, but to date she continues to enjoy her independence. Her story is a familiar one. Many people have spent their lives in institutions and it is only in recent years that 'the system' has allowed or encouraged them to live like ordinary people. For a large number of those people, the change of philosophy has come too late, and nurses often struggle with their consciences over whether it is kind to habilitate people of their advanced age who have been institutionalised all their lives. Each case has to be carefully considered on its individual merit, and age alone should not preclude their opportunity. Staff are often surprised that, as in Edna's case, life can begin at 70.

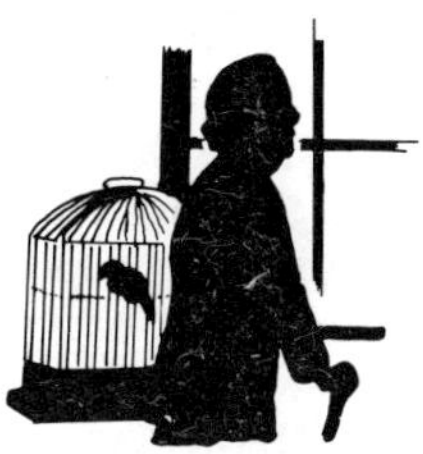

3 Incorrigible Kate

HISTORY

Kate was born in 1960. She was the second of three children, and the only girl. Her parents were both highly intelligent people, her father being a university professor, and her mother a schoolteacher. At the age of 2½ years, Kate suffered meningitis (inflammation of the meningeal coating of the brain). She had a high fever and was critically ill. She survived the initial illness, but was left hemiplegic, (partial paralysis of one arm and one leg) and developed epileptic fits. Damage to the brain only slightly impaired her intellect, but as she grew up, Kate became extremely frustrated by her inability to keep up with her brothers, who both attended university. Although Kate was very articulate, the conversation within the home often left her out of her depth, and she began to feel that she had failed in her family's expectations. She attended several ESN (Educationally Sub-Normal) schools, where she reached a reasonable standard of literacy, and became quite deft with the sewing needle despite her contracted right hand and arm.

The term 'educationally sub-normal' school has now been replaced by 'special school'

When Kate left school, the real problems began. Her epilepsy grew more severe, and her frustrations and continual striving to compete with her brothers (who were extremely understanding with her) caused Kate's behaviour to become very erratic and unpredictable. Temper tantrums in the home became an almost daily occurrence. Ornaments were smashed, and there was perpetual turmoil. Kate was accepted and expelled from every day facility in the area until the family were almost at breaking point. She was referred to a consultant psychiatrist in mental handicap, and a home assessment was carried out by the community nurse. Her mental handicap was not severe enough for hospitalisation to be considered, and yet no other establishment, day or residential, had managed to cope with her behaviour. Her father, by this time, had angina, and her mother was on the verge of a nervous breakdown. It appeared to them that they were being punished for their devotion to their daughter and there was no solution.

ADMISSION TO THE HOSPITAL

Finally, the situation reached crisis point, and Kate was admitted to the local mental handicap hospital, despite the view that it was not appropriate, just to give her parents the breathing space they so desperately needed. She was to stay for four weeks. Everybody was concerned about what her reaction would be to being admitted to a ward where the residents were much more handicapped than she was. It was felt that she would have no peers, or people to communicate and form relationships with on her own level, and that this would add to her frustrations and aggression.

Kate came quite willingly to the hospital, having had it explained to her that her parents were in need of a rest, and that she could have a 'kind of holiday' at the same time. Much to everybody's surprise, she settled into the ward very happily, and apart from wanting to telephone her parents every day, appeared to enjoy the change of environment.

It was not anticipated that any constructive programme of treatment could be carried out in such a short time, and the staff at the mental handicap hospital had only considered providing a 'hotel' facility for Kate to relieve the crisis at home. However, she achieved a very comfortable rapport with the nursing staff, and even befriended some of the residents. She began to talk spontaneously about her frustrations, and feel remorse for the anxiety she had caused her parents.

The informal psychotherapy which Kate received was quite unplanned, but the assessment of her epilepsy and anti-convulsant regime was intentional. Her fits were charted, and an electro-encephalogram carried out. This is a means of studying the electrical activity in the brain, which can sometimes be interpreted to indicate the type of epilepsy, and the appropriate drug regime to control fits.

At the end of the four weeks, it was generally felt that the hospital had something to offer Kate after all. At home she was a miserable failure, in hospital she was 'king pin'. Instead of feeling a failure, her obvious superiority in ability and intelligence on the ward gave her the very lift she needed. She was less frustrated with herself, as she became aware of the severe limitations of the other residents.

A case conference was called, and it was decided that Kate's temporary care should be extended, with a view to minimising her behaviour problems, and helping her to overcome her frustrations. Her parents, although still very devoted to her, were really anxious for her to 'grow up' and grow away from them somewhat. They felt stifled by her, even when she was behaving well. Every day of their lives, their holidays, their limited social life – Kate expected, indeed demanded, to be included. Her stay in hospital had been quite a new experience for them, because she actually stayed there. The staff did not reject her, she did not get expelled, her parents felt confident that they could relax and enjoy being together without Kate, knowing she was safe and happy. They felt strongly that it was time Kate started to develop friendships of her own, something she had never managed to do. Her parents were quite right, but did not know how to achieve their expectations. Their daughter was physically a young woman, but was still desperately clinging to them like a small child.

NURSING CARE

Initial stages

There were long discussions about, and with, Kate. She had sufficient intelligence to actually participate in her own individual care plan. With the ward nurses, she identified her own problems, and wrote them down. She found great relief and comfort in just sitting with the ward staff and analysing her problems. The ward staff did not become emotionally disturbed as was the case when she tried to talk to her parents.

Together, the nurses and Kate worked out the following care plan, with which she cooperated, with full commitment.

CARE PLAN

for Kate

Problem and aim: She has difficulty dressing unaided with one hand and needs an easy sequence of dressing and the addition of appropriate fasteners.
Nursing care: Provide a front fastening bra, elasticated waist clothing, casual slip-on shoes.

Problem and aim: She is impatient with her own slowness and needs time in which to do something. She must learn to appreciate any achievement, irrespective of the time required to accomplish it.

Nursing care: Make light of her slowness and encourage her to practise the manipulations that she finds difficult.

Problem and aim: She is intolerant of other people's needs and must try to see other people's point of view.
Nursing care: Ask her to assist other residents with her proficient skills.

Problem and aim: She has temper tantrums and needs to be taught to recognise the warning signs and seek counselling.
Nursing care: Respond to her request to talk about her problems, identify trigger points, and talk them through.

In addition to the care plan, Kate's behaviour outbursts were charted, together with her menstrual cycle and epileptic fits, to see if there was any relation. It was noted from this chart that often a bout of 'bad temper' happened the day after an epileptic fit, but there was no evidence that this was biochemical. Kate was always very depressed after a fit, and frustrated that their occurrence was erratic and unpredictable. It was often that this unhappy state caused her to flare up and overreact to quite minor incidents, out of sheer annoyance with herself.

Therefore it was apparent that Kate's epilepsy had a considerable influence on her behaviour. Her anti-convulsant drug regime was reviewed again, and constantly monitored in an endeavour to control the frequency of her fits. The nursing staff gave special attention to general health areas which affect epileptic people, such as regular bowel action, physical exercise, diet, and sleep patterns.

KATE'S BEHAVIOURAL CHART

31		X		X	X							
30				X	X							
29				X	X					△		
28		△			X							
27					X	X				○		
26		○				X						
25						X						
24				△		X	X					△
23		△		○		X	X					○
22		○	△				X					
21							X					
20			○				X	X				
19								X	○			
18						△		X				
17						○		X	X			
16								X	X		○	
15	△				△				X			
14	○								X			
13					○				X	X		
12										X		
11						△				X		
10			△			○				X	X	
9										X	X	
8	X										X	
7	X		○								X	
6	X						△				X	X
5	X	X		△								X
4	X	X	X	○			○			○		X
3		X	X		X							X
2		X	X		X							X
1		X	X		X							
DAY	MAY	JUNE	JULY	AUG	SEPT	OCT	NOV	DEC	JAN	FEB	MAR	APR

Key: X Menstrual cycle
○ Epileptic fit
△ Temper tantrum

Rehabilitation

Status Epilepticus: Series of fits following each other without regaining full consciousness

Unfortunately, despite these desperate attempts to reduce her fits, she went into status epilepticus on Christmas Eve, and was hardly conscious over Christmas Day or Boxing Day. A deep depression followed – Kate had been deprived of her Christmas, and a grand fling to demonstrate her annoyance was expected. Much to everybody's surprise, her depression melted away, and she expressed great concern for the nurses who had sat by her bed every hour, day and night until she recovered – because they had missed *their* Christmas!!

Kate was at last seeing things from another point of view! This breakthrough had to be very diplomatically acknowledged, so Kate and the nurses who had kept vigilance over her whilst she was having continuous fits were treated to their own private Christmas together later. Kate obviously received great satisfaction and joy from this, and her appreciation of their care was very obvious. She had learned something new about relationships – they had a two-way dimension – and it did not cost very much when what she was giving to the staff was her thanks.

Kate never really looked back. She still had epileptic fits occasionally, but her temper tantrums became more and more controlled. She learned to recognise when she was about to lose her temper, and above all, to understand why. She learned to reason with herself to a degree, and when she still felt that she was not in control, she would sit and pour out all her frustration whilst she screwed her paralysed hand with her good hand as she got it all out of her system.

Normally, it was not necessary for the nurse to participate – just to listen. Having voiced her feelings out loud, Kate usually solved her own problem and went on her way more composed.

Home visits became quite happy occasions that both Kate and her parents looked forward to, but she was encouraged to form other relationships, and get involved in social activities other than with her parents.

NURSING CARE

Planning discharge

Kate had been in hospital for five years before it was felt that she was finally ready for discharge. Her parents were delighted with her progress, but very hesitant and reluctant to risk removing Kate from the only environment which had proved therapeutic to her.

She herself was ambivalent about leaving hospital. Although she often talked about 'having her own home', she felt secure and confident in hospital, and a little anxious about people's expectations of her outside this sanctuary.

Again, Kate was involved in planning her future. She agreed to go to the Adult Training Centre outside the hospital daily, as a first step, and did amazingly well. After several months, Kate went for a trial 'holiday' to a local residential hostel, where residents were fully involved in everyday living skills – they shared responsibility for cooking meals, cleaning the house, and keeping the garden tidy.

There were 15 other residents at the hostel. Apart from the routine chores, Kate attended the craft workshop on site, and helped with the care of the animals in the menagerie. Her life was very fulfilling and meaningful. She was an important member of her community. She had her own bedroom which she took great pride in.

Above all, Kate learned to get her priorities right – her fits were the least important part of her life, not the most important any more.

Epilepsy is a disorder of brain function, causing convulsions and/or unconsciousness, due to idiopathic (unknown) or known causes i.e. birth injury, fever, brain tumour, brain trauma

Main types:

1 Partial seizure (previously termed 'petit mal') – patient momentarily ceases to be aware, then continues whatever he/she was doing. Often, the eyes roll up, or the patient stares into space, but does not usually collapse or lose consciousness
2 Total seizure (previously termed 'grand mal') – loss of consciousness accompanied by convulsions, see stages below
3 Jacksonian – seizure usually starts in one hand or foot, and spreads to the rest of the body
4 Myoclonic – brief spasm or shock-like contraction

Stages of total seizure:

1 Aura – a sensation preceding a fit i.e. a smell, sound, taste, particular movement
2 Loss of consciousness – the subject falls to the ground
3 Tonic spasm – contraction of muscles. Momentary cessation of breathing, often causing cyanosis
4 Clonic phase – jerking or convulsion of muscles, in which the tongue may be bitten, and incontinence often occurs
5 Recovery period

Treatment:

Basic good health care
Anti-convulsants
Intravenous/intra-muscular Diazepam (Valium) for status epilepticus

4 My fair lady

HISTORY

Annette was born in Uganda, where her father was assigned as director to an overseas branch of an oil company. The birth was normal, and for the first few weeks Annette appeared to be a beautiful healthy baby. However, long bouts of crying and screaming began to develop, and the usual milestones were not attained.

By the time Annette was two years old, it was quite obvious that something was seriously wrong, and the family returned to England to have their second child and to take Annette to Great Ormond Street Children's Hospital for investigation.

Physical signs of phenylketonuria:
Fair hair and skin
Blue eyes
Epilepsy

Annette was soon diagnosed as suffering brain damage caused by phenylketonuria. She was immediately put on the Minafen low phenylalanine diet, and closely monitored by the clinic. There had only been a couple of epileptic fits, but as her parents were very fair, she had lost what little colour pigmentation she was born with in her hair, and was now virtually white.

Her parents cared for her at home, with frequent visits to Great Ormond Street, until she was nearly four years old, by which time it was obvious that the diet was achieving nothing, and she was becoming very overactive.

ADMISSION TO THE HOSPITAL

She was admitted to the children's ward of a mental handicap hospital. Her programme of care commenced with a full nursing assessment. Although physically one of the smallest residents on the ward, the other children soon learned to avoid Annette, her teeth and her pinching fingers. Annette was a pretty child, and very affectionate with staff, but just as she had her arms twined firmly around the nurse's neck, she would suddenly bite into the shoulder, often leaving the marks of her teeth behind.

This unsociable habit deprived her of a lot of the affection and contact that she desperately sought. Her biting and pinching proved a very difficult habit to break, as Annette really did not seem to realise that her actions were painful and caused rejection. However, after a long period of perseverance and consistent response by the staff, she finally understood that her habit was painful and stopped it.

Annette did not talk, although she sang the words to nursery rhymes and songs quite clearly. If frustrated or annoyed, occasionally odd words would be expressed, but she could not be persuaded to talk outside these occasions. It was felt that she had learned to get along very well without conversation. When she wanted food, she dragged her mother or the nurse to the food cupboard; if she wanted to go out she pushed them to the door. She never took 'No' for an answer and persisted, getting progressively more bad-tempered, until she achieved her wishes.

NURSING CARE

Initial stages

Because of Annette's manipulative behaviour, her care plan was designed to increase her verbal communication and cooperation. Positive reinforcements for good behaviour, and a negative response for undesirable or demanding behaviour was the method used. Her positive reward was attention and affection, which she loved, but immediately she pinched, or bit someone, she was rejected and ignored.

CARE PLAN for Annette

Problem and aim: She demands attention by biting and pinching, an unsociable habit which has to be eradicated.
Nursing care: Give her normal attention and affection. When she bites or pinches, separate her from the group quickly and without emotion, and then ignore her for fifteen minutes.

Problem and aim: She picks holes in her clothing, and needs to utilise her digital dexterity more usefully.
Nursing care: Give her regular stimulation and activity, i.e. brick building and sorting, painting, plasticine play, lace and bead threading. Admire her nice clothing, and encourage her to appreciate her appearance.

Problem and aim: She does not speak and needs to be encouraged to do so.
Nursing care: Speak clearly and precisely to her. Repeat and encourage key words, such as 'drink, toilet, thank you, hello'. Reward her with affection when she responds by speaking. Do not respond when she pushes or points to her needs. Teach Makaton signs to be used in conjunction with the spoken word.

Her parents were very cooperative and keen to participate in her care programme, but Annette was so used to manipulating her family that they found it extremely difficult to show a negative response. When they tried, she would throw a temper tantrum, and they would feel so distressed that more often than not, they were driven to show a positive reinforcement in an endeavour to bring her out of the tantrum.

Rehabilitation

As Annette grew physically bigger and stronger, her behaviour became more of a problem to handle. Home visits were reduced to one night at a time, because Annette's sleep pattern became very disturbed when at home, and her parents had to relieve each other to keep vigilance over her. Strangely, sleeping was never a problem in the hospital ward, where she was ready to go to bed and usually slept well. Possibly the change of routine and environment caused her to be wakeful at home.

Her younger sister proved to be very successful with her; as she grew older, she took on the care of Annette during her home visits. Her sister was a very bright young lady who was very understanding and accepting of her sister, and sensibly asked for genetic counselling when she left school.

Annette's speech never improved beyond a few odd words, but she learned a more acceptable behaviour pattern, and basic self-help skills such as dressing, washing, toileting, etc. Her manipulative instinct was always just under the surface, and readily emerged if a new nurse arrived on the ward.

Her parents remained attentive, not only to Annette, but to the ward and the hospital as a whole. They were very supportive of all ward functions, and fully cooperative over Annette's care, about which they took a very realistic view.

Phenylketonuria is a metabolic disorder, in which the essential amino acid phenylalanine is not produced, or is produced at a very low level. The condition, untreated, causes brain damage, often with epilepsy, and disturbed behaviour patterns.

Diagnosis soon after birth is essential, and in this country a test for phenylpyruvic acid in the urine or blood has become routine on all new-born babies. If detected, a low phenylalanine diet is commenced and carefully monitored. (Too much phenylalanine is as damaging as too little.) There are several proprietary brands produced, the most common being Minafen, Lofenalac, and Cymogram. These preparations are unpalatable, and are often not readily accepted by babies and young children, and as children grow, it becomes difficult to monitor the 'forbidden' foods they eat.

There are several schools of thought about how long the diet should be given, and as this is a relatively new treatment, the evidence is not altogether conclusive. In some cases, the diet does not seem effective, or the parents find it difficult to manage and monitor, and it is abandoned early. It has been continued, however, up to school leaving age with varying degrees of success.

Invariably, because of the low pigmentation which occurs in this condition, if the child is untreated the hair tends to be in the blonde range, the eyes are often light blue, and the skin is pale and prone to eczema. The incisor teeth tend to be widely spaced, and the head circumference is often smaller than average.

The condition is caused by a single recessive gene, and siblings not affected by the condition may be 'carriers'. Genetic counselling is available and strongly advised for people with a family history of phenylketonuria.

5 Speak to me only with thine eyes

HISTORY

John was born brain damaged, and quadraplegic. The pregnancy had been problematic, and the birth protracted and complicated, culminating in a forceps delivery. The parents knew immediately that their baby boy was traumatised, but no one could assess how seriously until he was a few months old.

He had no voluntary movement of any of his limbs, his swallow reflex was affected, making feeding extremely difficult, and no speech at all developed. With time, his helpless limbs became contracted, and he could not be toilet trained because he had no control over his bladder or bowel.

Despite his gross physical handicap, John appeared to be very aware of his surroundings and familiar people. His parents cherished him and put so much effort into getting so little out of their son. Their patience was unlimited, and John quickly became the centre and purpose of their lives. He learned to communicate with them remarkably by the expression in his eyes. His mother knew him so well, she had little difficulty ascertaining her son's needs and emotions. John could look cross, happy, sad, hungry, thirsty, bored, pleased, too hot or too cold – all with his eyes. His facial muscles could give little help in conveying these feelings, but his eyes were very expressive.

John and his mother held long conversations, with mother doing all the talking, including what she thought John was trying to say, and he would very skilfully correct her if she misinterpreted his responses.

When John was eight years old, he was that

much wiser, and realised that he could manipulate and dominate his mother. He started having long screaming tantrums which lasted for hours sometimes, and his poor mother was becoming quite fraught. Finally, after a succession of tranquillisers and sedatives failed to achieve the desired calmness without drowsiness, his parents reluctantly agreed that he should go to a residential convent school for handicapped children. It was unfortunate that in the days of John's early childhood, there were no real community services for the mentally handicapped; with the professional assistance and support given today by Community Mental Handicap Teams, John and his parents could have benefitted considerably.

The convent school was used to dealing with handicapped children, but John proved far more handicapped than the children with whom they usually coped. However, with constant persuasion, they kept him until he was of school leaving age.

He achieved little, apart from the close relationships he built with the staff and other pupils. The school holidays, although looked forward to by his parents, proved traumatic and exhausting. John did not scream at school, but at home he screamed without seeming to draw breath whenever anyone came to the house, or the television was switched on, or anything else happened which diverted or diluted his mother's attention.

As John's sixteenth birthday approached, his parents were torn with anxiety about how they would manage him at home. The only placements which were available were not good enough for their son, and together they resolved to keep him at home – and cope. The 'coping' lasted about three months, before both parents were at breaking point. In desperation they agreed to a home visit from the psychiatrist and the nursing officer of the local mental handicap hospital. They told them of a new ward which was about to be opened at the hospital, for people of all ages, with physical handicap. The ward was small – twelve beds, and equipped specifically for non-ambulant people. A physiotherapist was to be based on the ward, and the staff given special training in communication skills.

ADMISSION TO THE WARD

John was offered the first place on this new ward, and despite his parents' ambivalence to hospital care as a permanent solution, they were tempted by the special facilities which would be available. The hospital was very near their home, which was another favourable point – and after much debate and soul-searching, they admitted John to the hospital, on a 'shared care' basis, which meant that he spent three out of every seven days at home. His mother was also encouraged to spend time on the ward looking after him; she got him ready for bed, and fed him often on the ward. This enabled the staff to observe and advise on John's relationship with his mother, and counsel her on the problem areas.

His mother found it extremely difficult to close the door on John when he screamed, and ignore him, but with encouragement and support from the staff, she learned to be less responsive to his unreasonable demands. John's screaming was obviously a problem which had to be solved, and although it was relatively easy to eliminate on the ward, even with his parents there, it was not as easy at home.

The staff decided that John was intelligent enough to realise very quickly the consequences of his actions, and if the parents found it too difficult to effect the consequence at home, then the nurses had to do it for them.

When all else failed, a plan was agreed, that John would go home as usual for his visits, but as soon as he began to scream, his parents would telephone the ward, and the Sister and a nurse would just come straight away and bring John back to the hospital with as little ado as possible. His parents' guilt feelings were less this way, and John soon began to realise that his visits home were very effectively cut short if he screamed. Fortunately this regime worked quite soon, as it was extremely difficult for the staff to keep it up. Screaming at home was never eliminated altogether, but it was reduced to a tolerable minimum.

The parents' biggest disappointment was that John could not speak, although, as already mentioned, his mother in particular was able to communicate fairly well with him. The ward practised various communication systems, and sign languages, including Makaton and Bliss Symbolics, but John could use none of them. His father was a very clever and practical man, and after studying carefully what little voluntary movement his son had, he built a 'buzzer bell' which could be operated very clumsily with his forearm. He then made pictures which illustrated John's needs, i.e. a cup of tea, a slice of bread and butter, the toilet, etc.

Makaton is the British sign language of the deaf often taught to non-speaking mentally handicapped people. It is a combination of finger spelling, lip reading, and, where possible, speech

Bliss is a collection of symbolic diagrams which a non-speaking person points to, in order to convey speech

This collection of cards were all shown to John in turn, and he would press the buzzer when the picture depicting his needs came up. Although rather laborious, especially as the collection of cards grew, it was quite a major breakthrough for John. It proved that he really could make preferences and decisions about what he wanted to eat, and wear, and he was obviously enjoying this small independence.

The Ward Sister had seen an Electraid Typewriter demonstrated at another hospital, and began to think that John could possibly use one if it had a special adapter. She told the parents about this machine, which was priced at £2000 without the special adapter which had to be individually made. The parents were so enthralled by the idea, they immediately started fund-raising activities, and in no time at all, the Electraid Typewriter, with several adapters to suit other residents on the ward, was installed. Such was the devotion and enthusiasm of John's parents. Their devotion was rewarded as they watched him make the first meaningful attempt to spell out phonetically what he could not say to them.

Although John did not progress beyond a few words and short sentences, his life took on a new meaning, and a lot of his frustrations were relieved.

His parents were a constant reminder to the staff of how important communication is, and how finding a way for handicapped people to express their needs very often solves other problems caused by frustration.

6 Mary, Mary, quite contrary

HISTORY

Mary was adopted when she was six weeks old. She was illegitimate, and her adoptive parents were enraptured with their new, raven-haired baby girl that they wanted so desperately. They had everything to offer a child. They were middle class, professional people, who viewed their parenthood very seriously. Mary grew into a beautiful toddler who won everybody's heart, and reached all the usual milestones until the age of two and a half years, when she began to give her parents cause for concern.

She stopped talking, became very withdrawn, and her habits became depraved. She was pre-occupied with her faeces, and seemed completely unaffected by her mother's obvious distress. Her parents began the long round of clinics and specialists, until Mary was finally diagnosed as 'autistic'. They were devastated.

Why should this happen to their lovely baby girl who was so bright and pretty and lovable? Where had they gone wrong? Mary went to a Rudolph Steiner School and received special training for autistic children. She progressed reasonably well, although she only spoke in monosyllables, in a very stereotyped fashion.

Her parents were still devoted to Mary, although by now they had a son of their own. They continued to press for the very best opportunities for Mary, even though her behaviour was such that they could not possibly cope with her living at home.

When Mary reached school leaving age, as often happens, there was no suitable establishment to continue the Rudolph Steiner special training, and after a long and traumatic ordeal, the parents relented and admitted their daughter to a mental handicap hospital.

Mary deteriorated steadily and consistently, and her parents were helpless to find a solution. She was now so withdrawn, that she lived in self-imposed seclusion. When the other residents were on the ward, she would go to the side room, and shut the door. When the residents left the ward for activities, the staff would coax her out, and she sat drawing at the table on her own. If anyone tried to talk to her or sit with her, she got up and left.

Her drawings were characteristic of her stereotype mind – all straight lines – even people were drawn in squares and oblongs, although colours were always correct. She would colour the nurses' dresses, and always leave a straight white apron. Spectacles were always very prominent in her drawings, and men always had clubbed feet. When she was menstruating, she coloured all her drawings bright red, but did not appear otherwise disturbed by her periods. She took to tearing her clothing, stripping, and smearing faeces. She screamed and made animal noises, and became very aggressive if anyone tried to distract her. Her adoptive parents were shattered. What could they do?

They toured the country looking for an establishment which they felt was right for Mary, but even when they thought they had found a place, she was not accepted. Eventually, they found a hospital which did not reject the idea of having her, and they felt confident that the programmes of care and training they were shown would be therapeutic. The problem was that the hospital had a catchment area, and their home was not within that boundary. In desperation, her parents put their beautiful home on the market and moved into the catchment area so that Mary could be accepted.

ADMISSION TO THE WARD

The receiving hospital sent a nurse to visit Mary and make an initial nursing assessment. That report left the receiving hospital in no doubt about the problems they were to be faced with.

The parents were invited to a multi-disciplinary case conference, where the staff were honest and realistic about what they thought they could and could not achieve for Mary. Her parents appreciated this honesty, and felt they had allies at last to help them and their daughter. They pledged their complete co-operation with any programme of care on which the staff would decide, and accepted that the plan would probably have to be changed several times to achieve any success.

Mary was escorted to her new home, and appeared completely disinterested and unaffected by her new surroundings. She immediately went to the dining room table with crayons and papers, and began drawing as if the environment had not changed. However, she soon discovered the difference; when the other residents returned to the ward at tea time, she searched frantically and in vain for a room to seclude herself. There wasn't one! There followed a long loud bellowing recital, and a few unfriendly slaps to innocent passers-by, and Mary spent the rest of the day crouched in the corner, with her fingers in her ears.

A week of patient observation followed, from which the nursing staff, together with the psychologist, drew up a list of Mary's serious problems, and decided to tackle them one at a time. Mary out-smarted them many times, and developed a few new anti-social behaviours every time they thought they had solved a problem.

Her parents visited regularly, but continued their utmost cooperation with her care programmes. If Mary had not 'earned' their visit they were content to spend a little time talking and listening to the staff about her progress or otherwise, and after a discreet peep at her, they would leave, confident that it was in their daughter's best interest.

Mary did not show pleasure in their visits, and after they had sat with her for a few minutes, she would pick up her mother's bag, hand it to her, and push them to the door. Their 'discreet' visits meant that Mary did not see them so often, and she actually began to appreciate their real visits and allowed them to stay a little longer.

CARE PLAN for Mary

Problem and aim: She strips off her clothing and needs to be taught to stay dressed.
Nursing care: Dress her in a full set of clothing underneath a strong suit, or under a restrainer harness. Remove the restrainer harness one hour before undressing for bedtime. Gradually increase the length of time without the harness.

Problem and aim: She is solitary and needs integration.
Nursing care: Encourage brief verbal and physical contact, first with the staff and then with other residents. Get her to serve and receive her meal plate from other residents and say, 'Thank you.' Allocate responsibilities to her such as laying the table or washing up.

Problem and aim: She tears her clothing and flushes them down the toilet, a habit which needs eradicating.

Nursing care: First plan – do not show emotion or annoyance, just replace the clothing and ignore her (did not work).

Second plan – Make her sew her torn clothing and wear it. Only replace the clothing which was flushed away (did not work).

Third plan – Encourage her to take pride in her appearance. Involve her in caring for her clothes, hanging them up in the wardrobe, ironing, etc. Admire her appearance (best result).

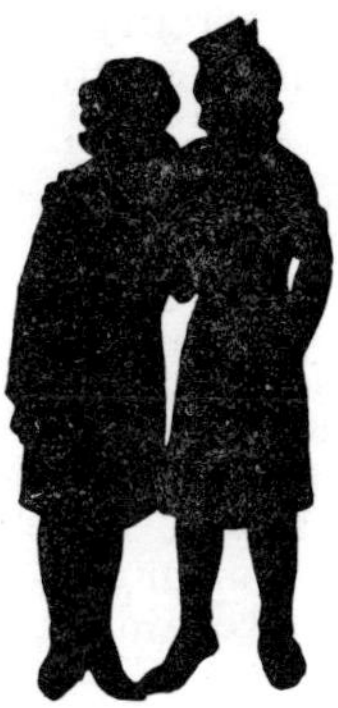

Her mother was a very smart attractive woman, and once Mary had learned to keep her clothes on, the staff started dressing and grooming her specially for her visits, much to her mother's delight. Mary began to really enjoy preparing for her visits, and amazingly, when she was dressed and groomed like a lady, she began to behave like a lady.

Her parents started to take her out for car rides again, and Mary sat in the car like the Queen, riding down the Mall. Despite this progress, she introduced her usual ritualistic element – as soon as she returned from her car ride, she strode straight to the bathroom, stripped off her clothing, and flushed all her underclothing down the toilet.

Getting her to keep her clothing on proved the most difficult task, and there were always periods of regression to stripping and tearing clothing whenever she felt annoyed or frustrated. It was difficult to understand how Mary could indulge in her obsession for abusing clothing, but enjoy wearing nice clothes for visits and functions.

She learned to tolerate other people's company reasonably quickly once she realised there was nowhere to escape to. At first she isolated herself in the corner of the room, progressed to sitting at a table on her own, and finally succumbed to sitting at the table with three other residents. There was one amazing occasion when the staff recorded with excitement, 'Mary sat voluntarily on the settee between two other residents this afternoon!'

Mary will probably always need expert care in hospital, but with the right kind of structure, her anti-social behaviour can be minimised to a tolerable level. At the age of 26 years, Mary now engages in more purposeful activity, and performs routine tasks on the ward such as laying and clearing the meal tables, and washing up. She can look and behave like a very sophisticated young lady. Her speech is still very monosyllabic, and her movements and expressions are stereotyped, although perhaps not so noticeably so since she is less angry and irritable.

Childhood autism is not in itself a diagnosis, but a term given to a collection of symptoms (syndrome). There are many conflicting theories about the etiology of the condition, with such diverse suggestions as metabolic, organic, or hysteric origin, or a reaction to emotional stress. However, it is widely agreed that it bears some resemblance to adult schizophrenia, and that the symptoms appear in children of all levels of intelligence. In broad terms it is a childhood psychosis, about which there is still much debate and research.

Common symptoms are:
Difficulty in forming or sustaining emotional relationships
Abnormal posture, grimacing, inappropriate expression of emotion i.e. laughing, crying, temper
Inappropriate use of personal pronouns i.e. refers to self as 'he' or 'she'
Pre-occupation with objects or parts of objects i.e. one wheel of a toy car
Resistance to change
Insensitivity to pain
Visual avoidance
Lack of inhibition and fear in the face of danger
Speech defects i.e. echolalia
Ritualistic habits and mannerisms i.e. twirling objects, and rocking to and fro
Stereotype movements of the body

Lack of visual perception i.e. demonstrated in distorted drawings

These children often look physically normal in a still position, and it is only their abnormal movements and expressions that make them noticeable in a crowd. A personal observation is that they are usually very attractive children, although there is no indication of why this should be so.

The usual pattern is that apparently normal healthy babies begin to regress, or merely cease to develop further somewhere between the age of 1–3 years. There is often a history of separation or emotional crisis within the baby's early years, such as illness or hospitalisation of the mother, another pregnancy, or some traumatic experience.

However, not all case histories of children with autistic symptoms reveal such an incident. Because of the withdrawn personality and often lack of meaningful communication, it is difficult to assess the level of intelligence, but autistic children often score well on the performance scale, despite their unwillingness to cooperate or communicate.

Complete recovery from autistic symptoms is not unknown. Mental handicap is often, although not always, associated with autism.

7 A rolling stone

HISTORY

Sybil's childhood and background were somewhat obscure. It was known that she had a twin brother, a sister and another brother. The family was split up and the children dispersed separately to children's homes when Sybil was still very young. She only had vague recollections of her family, but always a strong affection for the twin brother whom she hardly knew.

Her unstable childhood may have been responsible for her very disturbed adolescence. As a teenager, she was frequently involved with the law, and finally was committed to one of the special hospitals at the age of 18 years.

Special hospital: A secure hospital where mentally handicapped and mentally ill people with criminal tendencies are committed under the Mental Health Act

She spent the next 13 crucial years of her life locked up in the secure environment of the hospital, living with hardened mentally disordered criminals and social misfits. She learned the art of survival in this peer group, and became well educated in devious skills of the criminal and anti-social mind. She dabbled in stealing, violence, and suicide attempts – all of which were common practice in the institution where she lived.

By the time she was in her late twenties, she became depressed and anxious to escape the influences of her environment, and would ask to be locked in her room where she spent hours in solitude.

It was recognised that the special hospital was no longer therapeutic, or appropriate for Sybil, and vigorous attempts were made to find an alternative placement for her, but it is not easy to discharge people from special hospitals. Other establishments are often apprehensive about taking people who have a history of the kind of anti-social behaviour which caused them to be admitted in the first place.

Approaches were made to the mental handicap hospital in the area where Sybil's family originally lived, and finally a visit was arranged, and a nursing assessment made. Sybil happened to be locked in her room at the time the visiting nurse arrived, but cooperated with the interview, considering it to be her only chance of release.

She had become very institutionalised and reliant on the structure the special hospital regime provided. The transition was not going to be easy for her, or for the staff of the mental handicap hospital. She was only mildly mentally handicapped, and very proficient in her self-help skills. She kept herself meticulously clean and tidy, and took pride in her appearance. She could read and write quite fluently, and was used to intelligent conversation.

Sybil was not going to find any peers among the more severely handicapped residents of the mental handicap hospital. She was now 31 years old, but in many ways still the rebellious teenager who was admitted to the special hospital.

ADMISSION TO THE WARD

The transfer was arranged, and two nurses from the receiving hospital arrived to escort Sybil on the long 200 mile journey. Her departure from the special hospital was quite a heart-rending scene. The ward staff obviously had a great affection for her, and she wrenched herself from the tearful farewells of staff and other patients with some trepidation. They were the only people she had known for 13 years, and now she was about to step out into the unknown with two perfect strangers.

Her silence, apart from the sound of heavy swallowing, coupled with her expression of apprehension and bewilderment over the first few miles, gave some indication as to the difficulties Sybil's adjustment was to present.

When they stopped for lunch, she stayed glued to the nurse escorts, and relied on them heavily to assist her in choosing her meal. Once lunch was over, Sybil began to relax somewhat, and to talk to her escorts. She wanted to know all about the hospital she was going to, and mentioned several villages in the area which she amazingly remembered. She talked of her twin brother, and her desire to find him and her sister, with whom she had not had contact since she was a young teenager.

On arrival at the local hospital, Sybil was given a seclusion room as her own bedroom, to give her some of the privacy she was used to – the difference being that the door was not locked behind her. She was encouraged to arrange the room to make it comfortable and displayed her personal possessions. The nursing staff were very aware of the wide difference in the skills and abilities of the other residents in their ward and Sybil, and a careful programme of daily activity was arranged for her so that she had plenty to do which satisfied her capabilities.

NURSING CARE

Rehabilitation

There was also a considerable amount of time allocated to a planned rehabilitation programme. She had to get used to going outside the hospital, using public transport, shopping with new currency money, and feeling confident when doing these things on her own. It was not quite like teaching other mentally handicapped residents these social skills, because Sybil had done them all before, and was really very competent – she just lacked the confidence, not having had these experiences for 13 years.

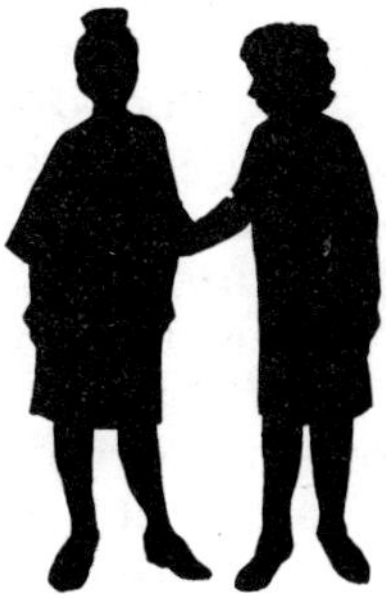

Sybil was able to participate with the nurses in planning her care programme, which she knew would prepare her for her ultimate discharge and open employment, the prospect of which she found exciting, but somewhat frightening. The lost years were beginning to show. She had to learn to live without the structure of a secure environment, to make her own decisions, and above all to accept the consequences of her decisions and actions.

At Sybil's insistence, eventually, her sister was traced. She lived at an address in a neighbouring town with her common-law husband and her daughter. Sybil wrote to her sister several times, but got no reply. She did not give up easily, and when a nurse offered to take her to her sister's house, Sybil wasted no time in writing to announce her intended visit. She had to find out for herself, whether or not she had a family who cared about her – whether she had any roots.

At the arranged time Sybil and the nurse drew up outside the sister's council house, and the nurse observed Sybil's mixed emotions of apprehension and excitement as she walked up the path and knocked on the door. There was no reply, and she knocked again. The nurse in the car caught sight of the curtains moving, and saw someone jump back from the window.

After Sybil had knocked several times, and it was obvious that her sister was not going to answer, the nurse called her back to the car, and tried to think of tactful excuses for her sister not being at home. Sybil desperately wanted to find somewhere or somebody she belonged to, to help her make it on her own. Her sister was obviously not going to be that anchorage.

A part-time job was found for her, on a farm collecting and grading eggs. She had been used to the outdoor life at the special hospital where she worked on the gardening party. Sybil enjoyed her job, but it did not provide her with the security and sense of 'belonging' she was seeking, and probably in a deliberate attempt to delay her rehabilitation programme, she started refusing to go to work on odd days for no specific reason.

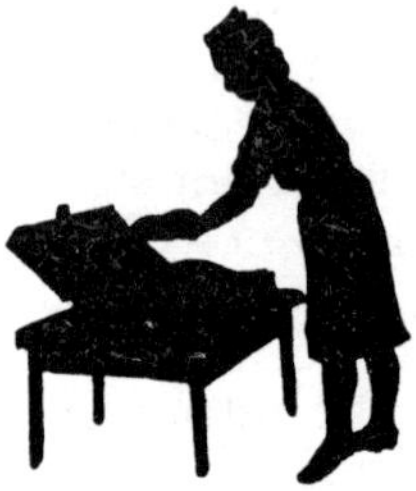

Her anxiety emerged in increasingly erratic behaviour. She was making sure that she would not be discharged into a world where she did not belong and had no roots. With reassurances from the nursing staff, Sybil agreed to go for a trial period to a social services hostel, on the understanding that the staff continued their interest and concern for her.

Whilst at the hostel, Sybil finally made contact with her sister, and it was to her that she went when she ran away from the hostel. After a week with her sister, she returned voluntarily to the hospital, rather disillusioned with the way her sister lived. She went back to the hostel, only to abscond again, this time with another resident.

This was to be the pattern of Sybil's life for several years. She was found several places in hostels and homes, but never stayed long enough to settle down. Her first point of contact was always the nurses at the hospital, who were the only people Sybil seemed to trust and look to for guidance, even though she seldom took that guidance.

She was not mentally handicapped to a degree that warranted her further admission to hospital, although that was where she wanted to live. After all those years of custodial care, she was unable to cope with her freedom.

She had grown to rely on the structure which organised her life for her, and relieved her of her responsibilities.

Sybil was a casualty of the system. Too intelligent to warrant hospital care, but too behaviourally disturbed to respond to the informal philosophy of most other establishments, her *insecurity* had been created by the *security* of the special hospital environment.

More and more, the nursing service is spreading out of 'hospital' and into community settings. If a community home had been available, staffed by nurses with a more structured philosophy of care, Sybil may have been able to continue the adjustment after leaving hospital. As it happened, she became a rolling stone, never settling, never feeling she belonged, never behaving in a responsible fashion.

8 The good life

HISTORY

Jake was one of two mentally handicapped brothers born illegitimately to parents of low to average intelligence. Both brothers were taken into care early, and at four years of age, Jake was fortunate enough to be fostered to a young couple who lived on a small holding with their own child, and one other foster child.

Jake was a pathetic little boy, physically well formed but very undersized for his age, and prone to self-mutilation. He would bang his face with his closed fist until red weal marks appeared which were very distressing for his foster parents, who were very caring people. Jake appeared to dislike all food, and mealtimes were a constant battle of persuasion. Even when his foster mother had managed to get a reasonable meal inside him, he would regurgitate it and retain very little.

He also wandered about aimlessly, and did not engage in any meaningful play. Knowing the problems the foster parents would encounter when Jake went to live with them, the maximum support was anticipated and arranged. The community nurse was heavily involved, in consultation with the psychologist, in drawing up programmes of care with which she could assist the foster parents.

Jake was rather a sad, solitary little boy, with some autistic tendencies, and this loving, understanding family were just what he needed. They were prepared to give unlimited patience, tolerance and love, despite his initial rejection towards them, and reluctance to become part of the family.

He was collected and taken to the special care class in the school for children with special needs daily, but when at home, he was taught, by a very slow process, to ride a pony, feed and help care for the variety of animals and birds on the small holding, and he could wander to his heart's content in the extensive grounds round the house.

His feeding problem reached a crisis point on several occasions, when he had to be admitted to hospital in a state of dehydration. It was carefully explained to his foster mother, who felt quite guilt-stricken at these times, that it is quite common for children who regurgitate to dehydrate themselves, despite their adequate fluid intake. There appeared to be no physical reason why Jake disliked eating, but he certainly appeared to receive satisfaction from regurgitating.

With perseverance, it was possible to get him to eat, so the community nurse decided the aim should be to prevent the regurgitation. After long discussions with the foster mother, the community nurse discovered that Jake needed his hands free to perform his ritualistic fingering routine in his mouth to initiate the regurgitation. If his hands were restrained in any way, he became so frustrated he then struggled free and banged his head and face – often until he bled.

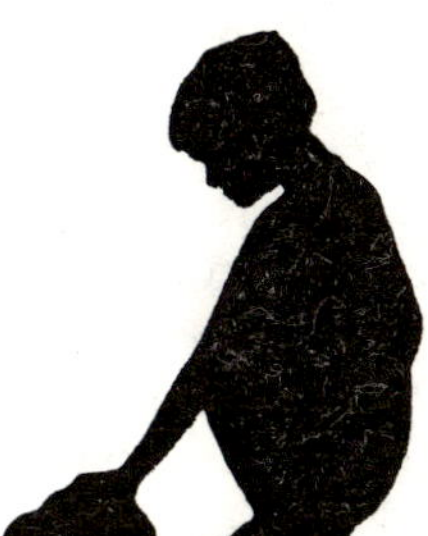

The problem was then, to find a way of occupying his hands immediately after a meal, in some activity which would provide sufficient distraction. Several play activities were tried, but Jake was not sufficiently interested in any form of play, and one by one, the programmes had to be abandoned and reviewed. Just as it appeared that they were beaten, the answer came in a flash. The community nurse arrived one afternoon to find Jake astride the pony, laughing hilariously, and clinging on for dear life, whilst his foster mother trotted the

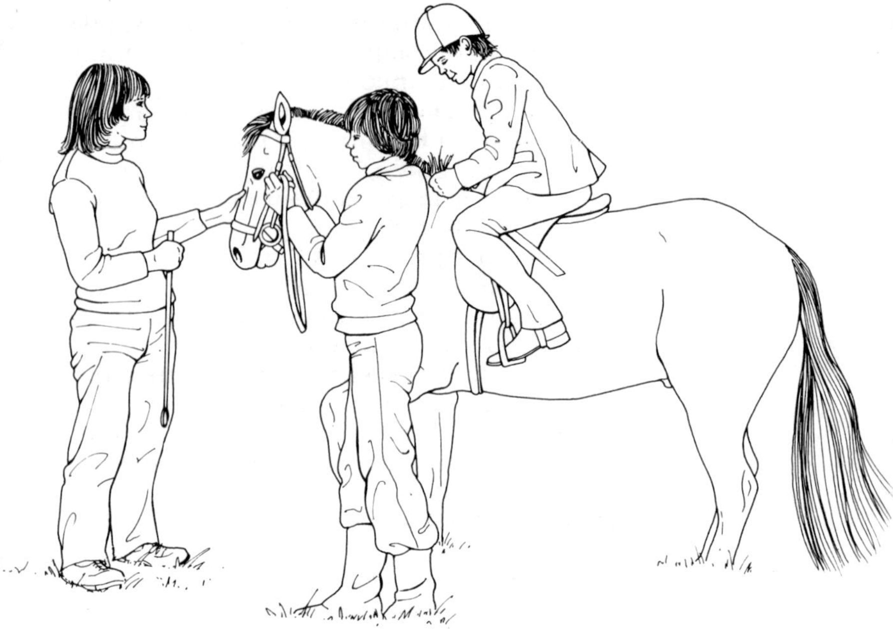

pony at jogging pace round the paddock.

Revelation 1 – Jake actually enjoyed this activity.

Revelation 2 – His hands were fully occupied holding on to the pony's neck!

'You can't be serious,' said his foster mother, 'That would be enough to make anybody sick, he wouldn't need to regurgitate.'

'Then what have we got to lose?' asked the Community Nurse, and together they carefully wrote down their plan.

Next day, Jake was given a very light breakfast, and the community nurse was there at the crack of dawn, to assist in the pony trot immediately breakfast was over – Jake was not sick, and after half an hour's pony trotting his digestion was well under way and he had forgotten he had eaten.

The same regime was followed at lunchtime

and tea time, and despite her thorough exhaustion from all the pony trotting, the community nurse returned in the evening to find Jake contentedly asleep on the settee in the arms of a very tired but happy foster-mum.

'It worked!' she crowed jubilantly. It then dawned on them that if they were to eliminate Jake's regurgitation, it could mean repeating this exhausting regime three times a day for a considerable time! However, after keeping it up religiously for a week, Jake began to put on weight and his cheeks became rosy – not with banging, but with health and exhilaration. The pony trotting was then very gradually diminished in length of time and frequency, and apart from the occasional relapse, the problem appeared solved.

Jake's relationship with the pony could not help but develop, and this proved a cure for his second problem – his self-mutilation. He had to 'cuddle' the pony to stay on his back, and the pony didn't try to cuddle him back! Jake didn't much like being cuddled, so this suited him fine.

The pony and Jake became firm friends, and a special bond of trust grew between them. Somehow this relationship seemed to relieve him of a lot of his innermost frustrations, and he learned to show real affection for the pony, an affection which he eventually learned to transfer to his 'family'. It was very fortunate that as Jake grew bigger and stronger, his head-banging diminished, because his new-found strength would certainly have injured him quite seriously.

Mentally handicapped children are often fostered, when their own families abandon them or are unable to cope emotionally with their care. Fostering often provides the best opportunity for normal development, and the child's full potential is likely to be reached more easily than in any other form of care.

The problems of attachments on behalf of the child and the foster parents have to be reconciled, and weighed against the long-term benefits of 'normal' childhood development.

Because foster parents do not have the guilt feelings of many natural parents, they are often able to participate more positively in behaviour modification programmes, and are not so vulnerable to manipulation by the child.

In Jake's case, his foster-mum was a 'super-mum'.

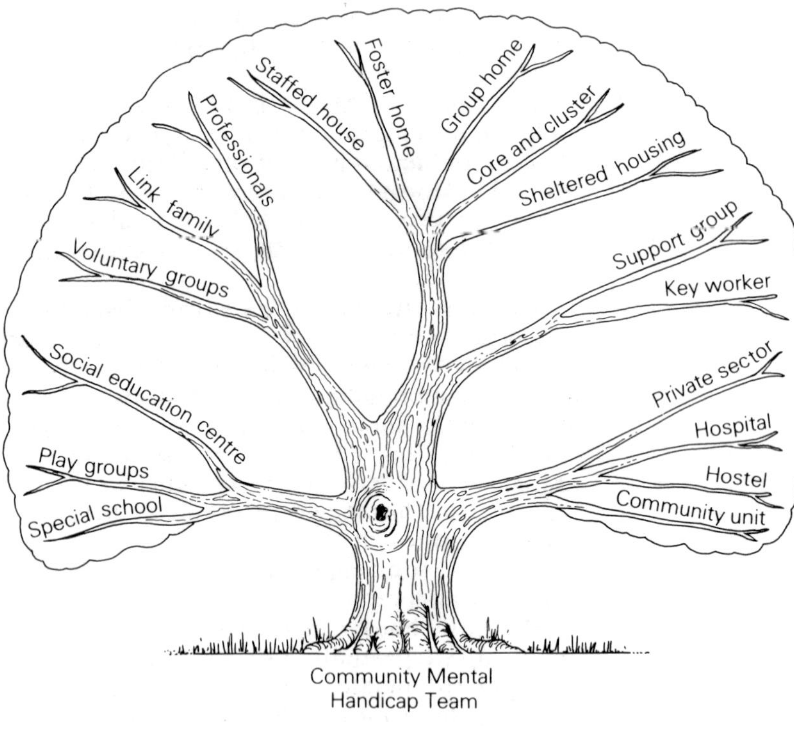

Services available to the mentally handicapped person through the CMHT

9 Summary

As you will have noticed, it is difficult to define specifically what the role of the nurse in mental handicap is. The needs of people with mental handicap are so wide-ranging, the nurse has to fill many different roles, according to those needs. The nurse certainly has to be resourceful, resilient, and often relentless.

It is important that every mentally handicapped person is respected as an individual, and that their views, preferences, and feelings are taken fully into account. Nursing care plans are vital to ensure that the service offered to the client is regularly reviewed, and that the type of care given does not stagnate. The care plan also ensures consistency of approach, and provides a continuum of development.

When considering a crisis intervention plan, to prevent self-injurious behaviour for instance, the nurse should first observe and chart the conditions under which the behaviour occurs, and the immediately preceding circumstances, i.e. does the behaviour always occur when a certain person is present, or after the radio is turned on or off? Unintentional reinforcements often occur and should be avoided i.e. the behaviour might distress the onlooker and prompt them to respond in a positive way by giving the person attention. If this occurs repeatedly, the severely mentally handicapped person learns that to get the attention he wants, he has to behave in this way.

Reinforcement of this kind is often difficult for the nurse to understand, because her response stops the self-injurious behaviour, in the short-term. In the long-term, however, it establishes an undesirable habit which is rewarding to the mentally handicapped person and the self-injurious behaviour takes on a more regular pattern. In behavioural problems of this nature, it is important for the nurse to enlist the expertise of the clinical psychologist, who can analyse the behaviour and suggest a step-by-step crisis intervention plan.

Whatever the type of care plan, it is very important that it is regularly and systematically reviewed and improved. Solving one problem does not mean you have achieved everything. There is always room for development, and other goals to be set.

In 1971 the Government produced a white paper called *Better Services for the Mentally Handicapped*. This paper advocated a whole new philosophy of care, and became the 'bible' to the carers of mentally handicapped people. Although superceded by many other important reports, the 1971 paper is still much quoted, and forms the basis of planning services for the future.

Objectives of *Better Services for the Mentally Handicapped:*

1 To extend and improve existing services and shift emphasis from hospital to the community
2 To invite greater sympathy and tolerance in the community and promote voluntary services
3 To give guidance to hospitals and local authorities on the development of services
4 To describe programmes of improvement and development already begun

Many of the recommendations in this document have now become standard practice, and as a result, the quality of life for the mentally handicapped person, and the support given to their families, has improved considerably. Nevertheless, there is no room for complacency. We still have a long way to go to achieve the rightful status in society for the mentally handicapped person.

Another important document was issued, in 1981, entitled *Care in the Community*. This paper brought about another revolutionary philosophy for mentally handicapped people. In short, it advocated that the majority of people with mental handicap should not be required to reside in 'hospital' and that various options in residential care should be encouraged. Some nurses interpreted this document as a threat to their profession, and envisaged a mass exodus from hospitals, and dole queues of redundant nurses.

In reality, what it meant was that by discharging the more able into other more appropriate forms of residential care, nurses would at long last be able to offer their undivided attention to the severely handicapped who require their expert care and treatment in hospital. It meant that the nurse's role could now be more clearly defined, and that mentally handicapped people with specific problems could be admitted to hospital for a planned programme of treatment/training, and hopefully discharged home like any other person going into hospital. Nurses, under these circumstances, could develop special skills which would bring rewarding results.

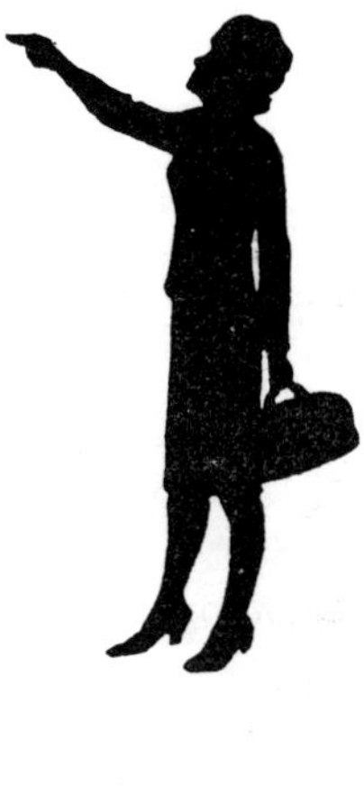

This new philosophy also meant that nurses could take their special skills out into the community, and help 'treat' mentally handicapped persons in their own home. Community care is now some way to being achieved, but again, implementing such a radical change has proved a slow, protracted process.

The National Development Team was inaugurated by the Government in 1975, and serves as a monitory and advisory body in standards of care up and down the country. They, and the National Development Group (now dissolved) have produced some very useful checklists and information pamphlets which the nurse learner would be well advised to acquaint herself with. They are included in the list of suggested further reading at the end of this chapter.

Mentally handicapped people are at last being recognised as an important group in society, and not just a section of third class citizens. Educating the public to accept the mentally handicapped as their neighbours has been no easy task, and the nurse is continually in a position to enhance public opinion and acceptance.

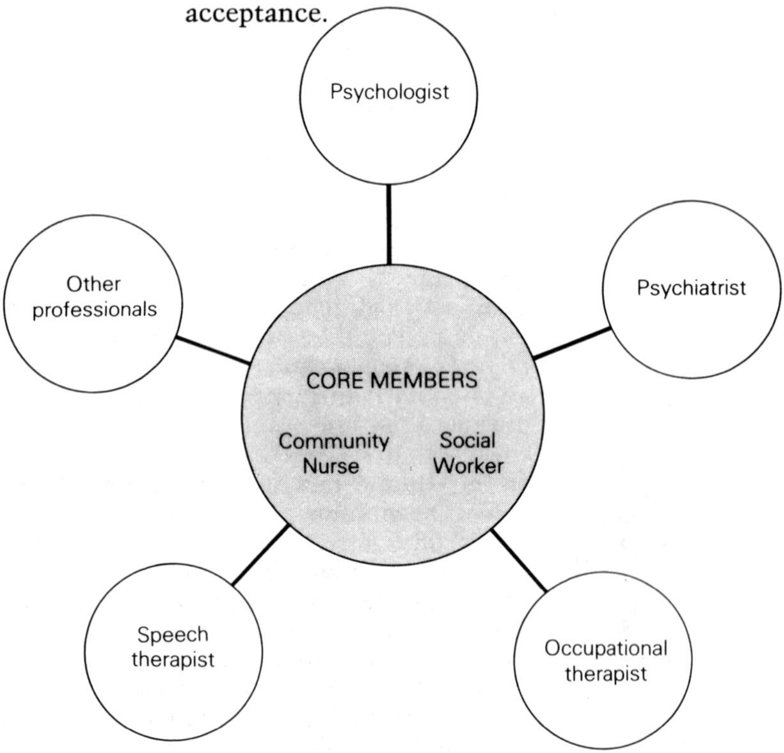

Community Mental Handicap Team

With the emphasis now firmly on community care, Community Mental Handicap Teams (CMHT) are in existence up and down the country. The role and structure of the teams vary slightly, but the original concept, as described by the National Development Group, is that each team serves a geographical area with a population of 60 000–80 000 people. The suggested structure is two core members – a fulltime community nurse, and a fulltime social worker. A psychologist, psychiatrist, occupational therapist, speech therapist and other professionals give part-time support to the teams.

The broad aim of the team is to keep a register of all mentally handicapped people in their area, and facilitate services to them. Regular reviews are organised to monitor the needs of the clients and their families, and to enable practical planning for the future. The core members are the co-ordinators of the teams, but are also practising members, offering their special skills where appropriate.

Some teams adopt the key worker system whereby the professional with the most appropriate skills acts as the main point of contact for each individual – i.e. where a mentally handicapped person's main problem is one of communication, the speech therapist may well be his key worker with the most input to that particular family. The CMHT should ensure that a family receives all the professional support and assistance needed, but at the same time, avoid too many people being involved, as families often feel confused and saturated if too many people are giving advice at one time. It is usually easier for them to relate to one person routinely.

The CMHT should have detailed knowledge of *all* available services and facilities in their area, and be able to introduce families accordingly. CMHT's often initiate Mothers'

Support Groups, 'drop-in sessions', sitting services, link families, play groups, toy libraries and many other innovative services to the mentally handicapped and their families. With all these facilities readily available, in addition to relief care, families are much more able and willing to cope.

However, it should not be taken for granted that every mentally handicapped person should permanently live with their parents. If we believe in the principle of 'normalisation', then we should accept that young adult mentally handicapped persons may wish to live away from their parents as most other young adults do. This is sometimes difficult for the parents to accept, and to find an appropriate alternative to the parents' home is a distinct problem.

There are many categories of 'group' homes, and it is now quite usual and possible for people with comparative handicaps to live in normal housing with the appropriate level of support. The more severely handicapped people may live in 'staffed' houses, where there is a 24-hour team of care staff, looking after three to five people. This is a very expensive form of care, but as it exposes the mentally handicapped person to all the normal experiences of everyday living, full potential development is more easily achieved.

Inability to communicate verbally is one of the more serious problems and frustrations of people with a severe degree of mental handicap. The frustration often gives rise to behavioural problems. It is important to distinguish between fundamental and secondary problems. If you only attempt to solve the secondary problem, a new secondary problem may well emerge to replace the one you have eliminated. So study your patient well. If he screams, or bangs his head, or tears his clothes, etc. – look for an underlying cause before trying to deal with the outward problem.

There are many alternative communication systems available for those who cannot speak. Makaton is a simple sign language which is fairly easy to learn, and most mentally handicapped people can master a few of the basic signs. The problem with Makaton is that it has to be learned, not only by the patients, but by everybody the patient needs to communicate with. Hence, it is important to include the whole family, and the friends of the patient, in the Makaton lessons.

Bliss Symbolics is another widely used communication system which is suitable for people with limited physical movement. It consists basically of a chart with pictures and symbols in squares, which the patient may point to. The symbols are much easier for the communicating person to understand.

With good speech therapy, it is usually possible to teach mentally handicapped people some speech, which can be supplemented by one of the communication systems. Unfortunately, there is seldom enough professional speech therapy available, and the nurse often finds herself making bold attempts to fulfill this important need. It is therefore very desirable for the nurse to acquaint herself with the more widely used communication systems.

Good physical health is very important to the mentally handicapped person, as often pain or discomfort produces secondary problems. How does the nurse know when a severely handicapped, non-communicating person is feeling unwell or is in pain? Make a list of the signs and compare them with the list below.

Signs of pain, discomfort and ill-health:

Pallor
Sleeplessness
Drowsiness

Crying
Screaming (headache, ear ache)
Limping (injury, corns, ill-fitting shoes)
Poor appetite (constipation, pyrexia)
Thirst (pyrexia)
Dribbling (toothache)
Shivering (pyrexia)
High colour (pyrexia)
Bruising/distortion (injury)
Difficulty in swallowing (sore throat)

Although good physical health is important to the mentally handicapped person, as with anyone else, it is perhaps an unfortunate anomaly that the 'caring' until recent years was considered to be the total responsibility of the Health Services. This inferred that the mentally handicapped person was 'ill' in some way. A more recent approach has been to include mental handicap under the auspice of the Social Services. For many years, this transfer of responsibility created a two-tier system of care, and two classes of mentally handicapped people, those with mild mental handicap who were cared for by the Social Services, and those with more severe handicap, who remained in hospitals.

Happily, these demarcation lines are disappearing, and Social Services and Health Authorities are now working together in many areas of the country to provide a comprehensive pattern of care for all people with mental handicap.

With the many alternative types of care available now in both the voluntary and private sectors, the service to mentally handicapped people is designed to accommodate their varying needs, instead of them having to adjust to a very restricted service as was previously the case. The service is now designed to consider the mentally handicapped patient as a whole person.

For this new comprehensive service, nurses might well, at some stage, gain a wider perspective than their solely health image, as the two major services draw closer together. The skills and expertise of the nurse will always be required however, and, to the mentally handicapped person with specific problems, the 'nurse' will probably always be the prime provider.

Whatever the future of mental handicap care, there is no doubt that mentally handicapped people are very rewarding and deserving to work with. The development of a more advanced and comprehensive pattern of service for mentally handicapped people is long overdue.

Further Reading

BRITISH INSTITUTE FOR MENTAL HANDICAP. 1981. *Ethical Implications of Behaviour Modification*, 2nd ed. Kidderminster: BIMH.

DHSS. 1981. *Care in the Community* (HC(81)9) *Consultative Document on Moving Resources for Care in England*. HMSO.

DHSS. 1978. *Helping Mentally Handicapped People in Hospital*. National Development Group for the Mentally Handicapped. HMSO.

DHSS. National Development Group Pamphlets:

1. *Mental Handicap – Planning together*. July 1976. HMSO.
2. *Mentally Handicapped Children – A plan for Action*. March 1977. HMSO.
3. *Helping Mentally Handicapped School Leavers*. May 1977. HMSO.
4. *Residential Short-term Care for Mentally Handicapped People*. May 1977. HMSO.
5. *Day Services for Mentally Handicapped Adults*. July 1977. HMSO.

DHSS. 1982. Mental Health Act-Amendment (HC(82)17). HMSO.

EASTHAM, R. D. & JANCAR, J. 1968. *Clinical Pathology in Mental Retardation*. Bristol: John Wright and Silver.

HMSO. 1971. *Better Services for the Mentally Handicapped*. Command paper 4683.

KIRMAN, B. & BICKNELL, J. 1975. *Mental Handicap*. Edinburgh: Churchill Livingstone.

O'GORMAN, G. 1970. *The Nature of Childhood Autism*. London: Butterworths.

SIMON, G. B. 1980. *Modern Management of Mental Handicap*. Lancaster: MTP Press.

WILLIAMS, C. 1981. *Behaviour Modification for Nurses*. Kidderminster: British Institute of Mental Handicap.

WING, L. 1976. *Early Childhood Autism*, 2nd ed. Oxford: Pergamon Press.

INDEX